HEALTH, BEAUTY
AND
A LONG, JOYFUL LIFE

(A modern paraphrase of Luigi Cornaro's
Discourses on the Sober Life)

Drop Kick Publishing
Atlanta, Georgia

DROP KICK PUBLISHING
Atlanta, Georgia

Health, Beauty and A Long, Joyful Life
Copyright © 2021

ISBN: 9798745350320

TABLE OF CONTENTS

Introduction...5

The First Discourse: On a Self-Controlled and Healthy Life.....7

The Second Discourse: Getting Rid of Sicknesses 22

The Third Discourse: Enjoying Happiness In Old Age.............30

The Fourth Discourse: Encouragement To Live To Old Age.34

About the Author 42

About the Editor...42

INTRODUCTION

Not being fond of long introductions, I'll keep this short. When Luigi Cornaro's story was translated from Italian to English it became very popular with people who wanted to live long, healthy, productive lives. But the translation was stilted, formal and not easy to read. Even so, many still benefited from following his advice, including myself. So I decided to re-write Mr. Cornaro's words in modern English. In transcribing his work this way, I was taken-up with him as a person and could almost hear him whispering to me as I felt the same zeitgeist that he felt in Venice more than 400 years ago.

When I was in my early 50's I was 40 pounds overweight. I had frequent heartburn, acid reflux, swollen and achy knees, painful elbow joints, a rapid heart rate, skin rashes and a host of other problems. I was also easily winded by the briefest of walks. But 5 months after taking Mr. Cornaro's advice, I had lost almost 40 pounds along with losing all of the above symptoms.

I'm almost 60 now, still in the superb condition and unless The Almighty has other plans, I intend to live until I'm at least 100. It's my hope that anyone who wants to do likewise will read this modernized edition and take it to heart.

Of course, before starting any dietary change it's a good idea to speak with your doctor but I'll wager that few doctors will disagree with this advice. Most will probably applaud it.

A word of warning though: Luigi Cornaro's style is definitely Old World. He goes on about things at some length, and sometimes repeats himself, which may irk the modern-day attention deficit reader a bit. But soldier-on and finish the book. It's not very long. If you read it with an open mind you'll enjoy the trip and quite probably add years and happiness to your life.

George Steffner
Atlanta, Georgia
October 25, 2016

The First Discourse: On a Self-Controlled and Healthy Life

Everyone agrees that whatever we do every day becomes second nature, whether it's good or bad. And after we do things for a while, we seldom think about what we do. We just do them. And when good people hang around with bad people, they often become bad people themselves. So I've decided to write about the lack of self-control.

Now we can all agree that the lack of self-control leads to gluttony and also that sober living comes from self-restraint. But because of custom, people who stuff themselves are thought to be right, while people who control their eating are thought to be mean and stingy. Most folks are so blinded and drunk that by the time they're 40 or 50, they start coming down with all sorts of painful sicknesses and diseases that leave them useless and unable to enjoy life. But if they had exercised self-control in what they ate and drank, they'd probably be healthy to age 80 and even further. And the best way to make this happen is to live simply and naturally, to be content with little, and to get used to eating only enough to support life. Excessive eating is what leads to sicknesses and death. I've had so many friends who were smart and had great personalities, who went from healthy to deathly sick simply because they didn't control their eating. If they had just learned how to control their appetites, they would still be alive today. It was a pleasure to enjoy these friendships but now I'm deprived of them and this worries me.

So to put a stop to this, I've decided to briefly write and show that we can stop being gluttons and start controlling our eating. I'm even happier to do this because a lot of younger people who understand what I'm saying have lost their own parents in middle life while I've kept my health all the way to age 81. They want to live as long as I've lived. Old age is the time of life when a person can exercise their wisdom and enjoy the lessons they've learned, sit quietly and reason out what we have learned. These younger people asked me to show them how they could live such a life and when I saw that they really wanted to know, I decided to write it down for them and any others who want to know how to stay healthy.

So I'll give my reasons for giving-up overeating and drinking too much and learning self-control. I'll show the way that I stayed healthy so that everyone will see how easy it is to do. I'll finish by showing what a great life I have from living a self-controlled life.

I had a long list of health problems that gave me problems and they're what made me learn to control my eating and drinking. I had painful stomach aches, heartburn and acid reflux, my joints were inflamed with gout. What was worse, I had a constant low grade fever with indigestion, and I was thirsty all the time. I figured the only way to get rid of these was to die.

So when I was between 35 and 40 I was miserable and had tried everything I could think of for relief but nothing helped. So my doctors told me that the only way to find relief, as long as I would stick to it, was to start regularly controlling my intake every day and that this was the only way to achieve good health again. They said that if I did this, I would see for myself that even though I had become weak and unhealthy, I wasn't so far gone that I couldn't recover. But they added that if I didn't start immediately, I wouldn't get any benefit from it and I might as well accept that I was going to die.

All of this made a huge impression on me. I was embarrassed at the thought of dying so early while at the same time miserable from all of these ailments. So I decided then and there to avoid sickness and an early death by eating correctly. When I asked my doctors how I should do it, they said that I should only eat and drink the kinds of food that are given to sick people, and in small amounts. I've got to say that they gave me these instructions earlier, but I didn't want to follow them and I kept stuffing my face and drinking heavily whatever I pleased. But this time, something inside of me clicked and I got the courage to follow what they said. So I started this new life with such determination that nothing since then has been able to change my mind. A few days after I began, I started to feel better. So I kept at it and in less than a year (believe it or not) all of my complaints were gone.

Since I'd recovered my health like this, I began to think about the power of self-control. If it could get rid of such awful sicknesses, I figured it must also be able to keep me healthy and make me strong. So I started figuring out what kinds of foods worked best for me.

First, I experimented to see if things that tasted good agreed with my stomach, because there was an old saying everyone knew that said, "Whatever tastes good must be good for you." But I found that this wasn't true because lots of things that tasted good made me sick. Seeing that the old saying was false, I gave up eating the meats and wines that didn't sit well with me and started eating only the things that didn't upset my stomach. I started watching not only what I was eating but also how much and ate only as much as I could easily digest. I never ate until I was completely full and began rising from the table while I was still a bit hungry. I followed the old saying which says, "To be healthy, you must control your appetite." Having mastered my appetites, I'll say again that I got rid of the problems that had seemed so incurable in less than a year. Not only that but I no longer had the yearly sicknesses that I had when I stuffed my face and drank excessively. I became very healthy and have stayed that way from then until this day. For that reason, I've never gone back to eating and drinking excessively.

The result of such a life has been that I've enjoyed and, thank God, still enjoy great health. Also, in addition to eating only foods that agreed with me, in amounts that I could easily digest, I've also avoided extreme heat, cold, extreme fatigue, interruption of my sleep and bad air. I also did everything I could to keep from depression, hatred and other extreme negative emotions that affect our bodies most. I've not always been able to keep these emotions away, but I've found that they don't affect people who live by the two rules of eating and drinking that I mentioned, which is to eat only what agrees with you and in reduced portions. Galen, who was a great doctor, said that as long as he followed the two rules, he hardly ever suffered from such sicknesses, and the few times he did, they didn't give him more than a day of discomfort. What he says is true and I'm a living witness of that fact as are many others that know me. They've seen how often I've been exposed to heat and cold and bad weather without getting sick. They've also seen me (because of bad things that have happened to me several times) quite worried. But these things didn't harm me much at all, while some of my family who didn't follow my way of living were very grieved at seeing me in expensive lawsuits that were brought against me by great and powerful men. They worried that I would be ruined as all are who don't exercise self-control. They were gripped with depression, which all who don't exercise self-control experience, to the point that they died before their time. But I didn't suffer like that at all because I didn't have the physical problems that they had. And to keep up my spirits I thanked God that He had let these suits come against me so that I could understand how strong my body and mind had become. I was also able to win against these powerful men with honor and I got a favorable decree both financially and also reputationally.

But I want to go farther and show how the self-controlled life also helps with physical recoveries from accidents. When I was 70, I was riding in a coach that was turned over while moving very fast. The coach was dragged a long way until the horses were finally stopped and I was shocked, bruised, battered in my head and body, and had a dislocated him and leg. When the doctors saw me, they decided that I would die in three days. But they did try to bleed and purge me to see if that would help. But I knew how pure my blood was from living the sober life for so many years, and I didn't let them do these things. I did let them set my arm and leg and let them rub me with oils as they said usually do. So without any other treatments, I recovered as I knew I would without any lasting ill-effects from the accident, which amazed my doctors. So we can see that people who lead sober, regular lives and don't eat too much will only suffer a little bit from mental disorders or physical accidents. On the contrary, I've recently seen that over eating and over drinking are often fatal. Four years ago, I agreed to increase the amount of food I ate daily by two ounces. My friends and relatives had been urging me to do this because they thought that I didn't eat enough for someone as old as I was. I told them that it was natural to be content with only a small bit of food and that I had been healthy and active all these years since I had been eating so little. I figured that as a man got older, his stomach got weaker and he should lessen his food rather than increase it. Also, I reminded them of two proverbs. The first said, "The one who wants to eat a lot should eat only a little bit because eating a little makes life long so that you end up living long and eat much." The second parable said, "What we leave at a big meal does more good than what we have eaten. " But what I said made them tease me about eating so little, and I didn't want to appear stubborn or seem like I knew more than the doctors, so to please my family, I agreed to eat two ounces more each day. I had been eating exactly twelves ounces of bread, meat, egg yolk and soup, and fourteen ounces of wine. I now I increased it to fourteen ounces of food and sixteen ounces of wine. Within eight days, I went from being happy and energetic to being sickly and depressed to where nothing could make me happy. By the twelfth day, I got a terrible pain in my side that lasted twenty-four hours. This was followed by a fever that lasted thirty-five days without letting up until everyone thought I was a goner. But I recovered, thank God, and I'm now certain that my years of eating and drinking correctly was the only thing that kept me from the jaws of death.

Orderly living is certainly a cause of health and long life. No, I'll say that it is the only true medicine and anyone who thinks about it for a while will come to the same conclusion. So when a doctor makes a house call to a patient, the first thing he prescribes is regular living and to avoid excesses. After recovering, if the patient continues to live this way, he shouldn't be sick again, and if a very small amount of food restored his health, only a bit more would be necessary to stay healthy, which meant that he wouldn't need a doctor or medicine in the future. And by following what I'm saying, a person would become their own doctor. And this would be the best doctor of all because no one knows their own body better than they know themselves. This is because by trial and error, a person may acquire a perfect knowledge of their own body and know the kinds of food and drink that agree with him best. These trials and errors are necessary since everyone is different. I found that old wine didn't suit me but that new wines did. After a lot of practice, I discovered that a lot of things that might not bother other people didn't work for me. Tell me where is the doctor that could have told me what to eat and what to avoid? After all, it was pretty difficult to figure out for me to find out for myself what was best by watching it for a long time.

It follows then that it is impossible to be a perfect doctor for another person. A person can't have a better guide than himself or any prescription better than the regular living that I've described. I don't mean to say that those who live this regular life don't ever need a doctor or that we shouldn't give him the respect he's due. We should call a doctor when we get sick. But for simply staying healthy, it's my opinion that we should consider this self-controlled, regular life as our doctor, since it keeps even weak people healthy and causes them to live well and hearty the age of one-hundred and further. It prevents them from dying of sickness or the corruption of their bodies but rather allows the natural decay which eventually comes to everyone. But only a few people discover these things because folks are for the most part slaves to their appetites and are without self-control. They love to satisfy their appetites and commit every excess. They explain that they would rather a short life where they can eat and drink like pigs rather than a long self-controlled life. What they don't realize is that the happiest people are the ones who keep their appetites in check. So I'd rather live a self-controlled life that will be long and productive. I wouldn't have even been able to write these words that hopefully will help others, unless I had lived a life of self-control. People who live uncontrolled, gluttonous lives say that no one can live the way I'm describing. To this I can only say that the great doctor, Galen, led this kind of life and chose it as the best medicine. Plato did the same, as did Cicero, Isocrates, and a lot of other great men of earlier days, along with many more I won't mention to avoid boring the reader. And in our time, it was Pope Paul Farnese and Cardinal Bembo, who lived long because of eating simply as I've described. And since so many people have lived this type of life (and are leading it now), it seems logical that anyone could do it, since it's really not that difficult to do. Cicero says that you only need be determined to live this way. Plato lived this way but admitted that in republics, men cannot do it because they have to expose themselves to many hardships and changes which keep a person from living this way. I can only answer that men who endure these things could bear them easier if they were self-controlled in their eating and drinking.

Now here, someone might say that a person who leads a self-controlled life where they were well, only ate a little bit of the simple food that sick people eat, has nowhere to turn for food when they become sick themselves. My answer is that whoever leads a simple and regular life can't be sick, or can't be sick very often. By a regular life, I mean that a person finds out how little food and drink is sufficient to supply their body's daily needs, and having done this, they then find the foods and drinks that suit them best. Then they should make their plans and adhere strictly to them, not being careful sometimes and self-indulgent at others. If they did it that way, they wouldn't be helped much. But if they are careful to always avoid excesses, anyone can do if they are determined. I can only say that such people can't be sick or at least not very often and then only for a short time. It's because of regular living that they destroy every seed of sickness. By removing the cause, they prevent the effect. Anyone who pursues such a regular and strictly moderate life doesn't need to fear illness because their blood is pure and is free from infections. It's not possible that they can fall sick.

Since such a life is also profitable and upright, it should be followed by everyone. And since it doesn't clash with everyday duties, it's easy for everyone to do it. But it's not necessary that everyone should eat as little as I eat, which is twelve ounces, and they also don't have to avoid the same foods that I avoid because of the natural weakness of my stomach. If you find foods that agree with you, eat them. Just don't eat a greater amount than the stomach can easily digest, even if it agrees with you. It's the same with drink. The only rule in this case is to observe is the quantity rather than the quality. But for someone like me who has a weak stomach, they should be careful of both quality and quantity, and eat only those things that are easy to digest.

No one should tell me that some folks live uncontrolled lives of gluttony that live to ripe old age. This argument is grounded in uncertainty and hazard and such cases are rare. Folks shouldn't, because of these exceptional cases, choose to stuff their faces with foods that taste good but aren't good for them. Whoever trusts that he is healthy enough to eat and drink this way should expect to suffer by doing it and live in constant danger of disease and death. So I say that even someone who is weak and sickly who leads a strictly regular and sober life is surer of living long than a strong person who lives carelessly and irregularly. If people intend to live long and be in good health, and then die without sickness of body or mind, but by mere dissolution (closing down) of the body, they must submit to a regular life in which they abstain from excess of food and drink. Such a life keeps the blood clean and pure, and allows no burping to come up from the stomach into the head. The brain of such a person enjoys constant serenity. Such a person can soar above the low and groveling concerns of this life and dwell more on the comforting and satisfying wonders of Heavenly things. Such a person then can see the brutality of the excesses that people fall into, which bring them misery not only here but in the hereafter, and they can have the comfort of looking forward to a long life with the knowledge that through God's mercy, they have said no to the paths of vice and excess, never again to say yes to them, and through the merits of our Savior Jesus Christ, to die in His favor. Such persons don't allow themselves to be discouraged by thoughts of death, since they know that death will not attack them with violence or by surprise or with sharp pains and feverish sensations, but it will come upon them with ease and gentleness. Like a lamp that has run out of oil, they will pass gently and without any sickness from this earthly mortal life to a heavenly eternal life.

Some sensual unthinking folks say that a long life is no great blessing and that anyone who is over seventy-five can't be said to be living. But this isn't so at all as I shall show you, since it's my sincere wish that everyone would live to my age so that they might enjoy this most enjoyable period of life. It is more desirable than all others.

I'll give a list of my recreations and the fun which I find at this stage of life. A lot of people can verify how fun my life is. First, they see how healthy I am in both body and mind. I can mount a horse without help, climb stairs easily and I've got a good-natured, happy personality. My mind is always unworried and it's filled with joy and peace. They can also attest to how I pass the time each day. I'm never bored. I pass the hours happily, talk with level-headed, intellectual men, and when I'm not with them, I always have a good book to read. And when I've read as much as I like, I write, trying in this and in other things to be of service to others. And I do these things with the greatest of ease, living in a pleasant house in the most beautiful quarter of this noble city of Padua. Besides this house, I have my gardens which are supplied with pleasant streams where I always find something fun to do. And none of these activities are any less fun due to the failing of any of my senses. For all of my senses are, thank God, perfect, particularly my sense of taste which is sharper now with simple foods than it was back when I ate the fanciest of foods and led an undisciplined life. And I'm not uneasy when I change beds. I'm able to sleep everywhere soundly and quietly, and my dreams are pleasant and delightful. I also take in undertaking a task for the state, namely the draining and improving of uncultivated ground, which began a long time ago but one that I never thought I would live long enough to see it completed, but I have, and I was even able to assist the work for two months in the marshes during the summer heat without ever suffering from any fatigue from it. This is because of the orderly life I always lead. These are some of the things I do as an old man. And I value doing these things even more than I value my old age or the age of younger men because, being freed by God's grace from the worries of the mind and aging of the body, I no longer experience any of those disagreeable emotions that rack so many young and old men because they have lived carelessly and eaten and drunk excessively, don't have their health, strength, or any true enjoyment.

And if it's all right to compare little things to big things, I'll also say that since I've led such a sober life, I have, at the age of eighty-three, been able to write an entertaining comedy that is full of innocent laughter and pleasant jokes.

I have still another comfort that should be mentioned, which is seeomg a kind of immortality in a succession of descendants because whenever I come home, I find waiting for me not one or two but eleven grandchildren, the oldest of them being eighteen and all of them the children of one father and mother and all blessed with good health. Some of the youngest ones, I play with, while I consider the older ones to be my companions. Nature has given them good voices and I enjoy listening to them sing and play different instruments. And I sing with them myself because I have a better voice now that is clearer and louder than any that I have had at any other time in my life. Such is the fun I am having in my old age.

So you can see that life I lead isn't gloomy but cheerful. I wouldn't trade my life and my gray hair with a young man's who was full of health and living an undisciplined life, because I've learned that this kind of person is daily subjected to a thousand different ailments and even death. I think back on the way I lived my early life I remember how foolish young men are and how they feel bulletproof. And due to their lack of experience, they are over-confident in their expectations. So they often expose themselves rashly to all sorts of dangers and, forgetting common sense, engage in the slavery of sexual immorality as they try to satisfy all of their appetites, not realizing that they are fools and that they are rushing toward the very thing that they want to avoid, namely sickness and death.

And are the two great evils of such a free life. On one hand it's troublesome and painful, and on the other, it's dreadful and unsupportable, especially when you think of all of the other errors that mortals can fall into in this life, as well as on the vengeance that God in His justice will take on sinners. I thank God Almighty that, as an old man, I am immune to these torments, the first one being that I can't get sick because I've removed everything in life that causes illnesses by living a regular life of moderation. The second torment that I don't have is the fear of death since by so many years of experience I have reasoned that it's silly to fear that which can't be avoided, not to mention the fact that I firmly expect some consolation from the grace of Jesus Christ when it's time for me to finally move on.

But although I'm aware that I must, like everyone else, reach that time, it's so far away that I can't make it out yet because I know that I'll simply pass away some day, since because of my self-disciplined life, I've avoided all of the other ways to die and prevented the tissues of my body from taking me out any other way than that which I expect in this mortal body. I'm not so naïve that I can't see that as I was born, and that I'll eventually die. But the natural death I'm talking about doesn't overtake a person until they've lived a long, long time. And even then I don't expect to be in pain and agony when I go, as so many have when they've died. But by God's blessing, I reckon that I will be around for a long time and that I will enjoy health and good spirits and enjoy this beautiful world which is beautiful to those who know how to make it beautiful. But its beauty can only be seen by, from wise living, they who enjoy sound, healthy, bodies and minds.

Now since this sober and moderate way of living brings so much happiness and if the blessings that come with it are so stable and permanent, I beg everybody who can think well to grab onto this valuable treasure, this long, healthful life, a treasure that's greater than all other worldly blessings that we should seek out. For what good is wealth and plenty to a person who has a weak, sickly body? This is the divine sobriety that God likes, this friend of nature, daughter of reason, sister of all of the other virtues, friend of self-controlled living ... modest, polite, content with little, regular, and the perfect companion. From this sobriety, as from any proper source, come life, health, cheerfulness, a good work ethic, learning, and all of the actions and accomplishments that are worthy of noble and generous minds. The laws of God are in sobriety's favor. Being over-fed, being excessive in eating, drinking, having unneeded substances in the body, diseases, fevers, pains, and the dangers of death vanish in her presence, just as the mists vanish before the sunrise. Her beauty attracts every friendly mind. Her influence is so dependable that it promises a long and agreeable life. And lastly, she promises to be a mild and pleasant guardian of life, teaching how to ward off the attacks of death. Strict sobriety in eating and drinking renders the senses and understanding, makes the memory strong, and makes the body lively and strong, with regular and easy movements. The soul feels little of her earthly burden and experiences much of her natural liberty. People in this state enjoy a pleasing and agreeable harmony, since there is nothing in the body to disturb. The blood is pure and runs freely through the veins while the temperature is mild and not fevered.

The Second Discourse: Getting Rid of Sicknesses

My writing on a sober life has done what I had hoped, namely to be of service to many persons that were born with less than healthy bodies or, the other persons who have lived far too extravagantly and have found themselves in bodily trouble. I would like to be of service to those who were born with good health but because of excessive eating and drinking, are attacked with all sorts of pains and diseases like gout, sciatica, liver and stomach complaints when they are only fifty or sixty. They wouldn't be subject to all of these if they lived a strictly self-controlled life and if they did control themselves in this way, they would greatly lengthen their lives and live in greater comfort. They would be less irritable and less likely to be impatient with inconveniences and annoyances. Personally, I had a very irritable disposition and I was very hard to live with. But now for a long time I've been easy going. With hindsight, I can see that a person that's controlled by their passions and emotions is no better than an insane person.

The person who has bad health may, by thinking things through and becoming self-controlled, live to a ripe old age and be in good health as I have. It seems impossible at first that someone like me could live past forty, but here I am now, at eighty-six ... forty-six years further than I thought I would live. During this long time, I've kept all of my senses perfectly. Even my teeth, voice, memory are perfect. Even more, my thinking is clearer now than it ever was. None of my abilities decrease as I age and it's because as I age, I decrease the amount of solid food I eat. This is necessary since nobody lives forever, and as the end draws near, a person is brought so low that they are able to live for twenty-four hours simply on the yolk of an egg and a few spoonfuls of milk with bread. More than this would probably be painful and shorten life. In my own case, I expect to die without any pain or sickness and this is an important blessing.

But it's expected of any who lead a self-controlled life, whether they are rich or poor. And since everyone should want to live to an old age, everyone is duty bound to do their best to live a long time. But it's impossible to do without strict self-control in eating and drinking. Some say that a lot of people live to a hundred years even though they stuff themselves and drink to excess and these folks think that they can do the same thing. But this is wrong in two ways: first, not one in fifty-thousand can get to that happy state, and second, at the end of their lives, such over-indulgence will lead to sickness that carries them off. They can't be sure of ending their days on earth otherwise. The safest way to a long and healthful life is to be sober with a strict control of how much they eat. And this is easy to do. History tells us of lots of folks who lived with self-control and currently we can find many such folks. I am one of them. All humans can reason things out, so we should be the master of all of our actions.

The sobriety I've mentioned is boiled down to two things: quality and quantity. The first involves avoiding foods and drinks that disagree with our stomachs. The second involves eating only so much as our stomachs can easily digest. Everybody over the age of forty should be able to figure this out. And everybody that follows these two rules is living a regular and sober life. And the great thing about such a life is that your blood becomes pure, which causes you to be unaffected by too much heat or cold, or too much fatigue, the lack of rest, or similar things. Someone who lives in this way can move through all of these situations without harm to themselves, since the bodies of folks who observe these two rules cannot be corrupted or catch diseases (which cause early death). Everyone should follow these rules, and if they don't they expose themselves to disease and death.

And the people who follow the two rules in diet, which gives them good health, can, by being in extreme heat, cold, fatigue, etc., find themselves indisposed for a day or two, but they don't need to fear anything else.

Some folks who are up in years are reckless in the way they eat and drink and say that it makes no difference to them, so they stuff themselves and drink heavily. Such people are ignorant of how the body works or they are simply gluttons. And I'll say that they are in poor health and usually sick, irritable and full of problems. There are others who say that they must eat and drink a lot so that they can stay warm, since it gets harder to as they age. These say that it's their duty to stuff themselves with food that tastes good. They say that if they controlled their intake, they would shorten their lives. Thousands of people use this excuse but it's my opinion that they are deceiving themselves. I speak from experiences as well as observing others. The simple fact is, large quantities of food can't be digested by old stomachs. We get weaker as we age and the elimination slows down, while the body's heat decreases. And all the food in the world wouldn't remedy these things but would instead bring on fever and sicknesses. So don't be afraid of shortening the life by eating a little bit. I am strong and healthy and full of good spirits and I don't have aches or pains even though I live on very little food. Regarding food, if this method suits one person, it will suit another. Whenever people get sick, they reduce their food. So if by reducing their food, they can recover from serious illnesses, a reasonably slight increase after the sickness will support the body if it's healthy. Try it for a few weeks and see if you have good results.

Other people say that it's better to suffer three or four times a year from ailments than to suffer all year long by starving. They say that the effects of excessive eating and drinking can be removed by a few days of self-denial. But if they normally eat and drink to excess, they can't have enough strength to get over these sicknesses with temporary self-control and some day one of these sicknesses may take them away for good. They shorten their lives with this kind of living as much as self-controlled people lengthen their lives.

Others say that it's better to live a shorter life with gluttony and drunkenness than a long life that is self-denied. But a long life is surely more valuable. Folks who understand things do value long life. Long life is a gift from God and should be prized and any who don't prize it are a disgrace to their fellow humans. Their death is a service to humanity. Again, some folks, seeing that they are getting weaker as they age, can't be convinced that they should decrease their quantity of food. Rather, they increase it and since they can't digest so much food two or three times a day, they decide to eat a lot, but only once a day. But it's still no use to eat a lot this way for the stomach is overloaded and the food isn't fully digested and turns into garbage that poisons the blood and is fatal to such a person long before their time. I've never seen an old person who was healthy and lived like this. Now all of these folks I've described would live long, happy lives as they aged if they would decrease the quantity of their food and ate more frequently with only a little bit at a time. Old stomachs just can't digest a lot of food. People of this age are like children again and must eat small amounts often in a twenty-four hour period.

Oh three times holy sobriety, so useful to people because of what you cause in them. You prolong people's lives and thereby improve their understanding. With this understanding they can avoid the problems of immorality which war with people's reason. You also free him from the terrible worries about death. We should be greatly indebted to you since by you we enjoy this beautiful world, which is really beautiful to the ones whose sensibilities haven't been dulled by excesses, and whose minds haven't been attacked by immorality! I never really saw how beautiful the world was until I got older. When I was young, my health was damaged from excessive living, so I couldn't see and enjoy how beautiful the world is. Additionally, what a happy life I have now that my body is so healthy, now that plain bread tastes so much better than fancy food used to taste. In fact, I taste sweetness in plain bread because of the good appetite I always have. I'd be afraid of living excessively now that I see the need of living moderately. I know that pure bread is the best food and as a person lives a self-controlled life, they never need to add fancy sauce food since a good appetite causes food to taste wonderful. Also, I've seen that while I used to eat twice a day, now that I'm much older it's better to eat four times a day, while decreasing the quantity as the years increase. I do this from experience. My spirits are brisk especially after eating, and they are never oppressed by eating too much to the point that I enjoy singing a song before I sit down to write.

And I never have any problem writing after eating my meals. My understanding is clearer, I'm never drowsy and the food I eat is too small in quantity to cause me acid reflux or burping and heartburn. Oh how great it is to an old man to eat small amounts. So I eat just enough to keep body and soul together. These are the things I eat: bread, breaded cutlets, egg (just the yolk), and soups. The meats I eat are veal and mutton. I eat all sorts of poultry along with fish from both the sea and the river. Some folks are too poor to afford such foods but they can still eat well on bread (made from wheat meal which contains a lot more nutrients than bread that's made from fine flour), breaded cutlets, eggs, milk and vegetables. But although people may eat nothing but these good foods, they should still be careful not to eat more than their stomachs can easily digest, never forgetting that over-filling the stomach injures even more than eating unsuitable food. I'll say again that anyone that doesn't break the two rules, namely, quantity or quality, will die not from sickness but from simply running out of steam unless of course they've inherited some disease. This kind of disease is rare, but a self-controlled diet will be of great service even to that problem.

Oh what a difference there is between a regular, self-controlled life and an irregular, out-of-control life! One gives you health and long life while the other produces disease and an early death. I've lost so many dear relatives and friends because of their excessive habits. If only they had listened to me they might still be full of life and health. This makes me even more determined to work hard telling people how my kind of life is beneficial. Here I am, an old man yet still full of life an joy, happier than at any other time in my life, surrounded by lots of comforts, not the least of which are my eleven grandchildren, all of them with fine minds and agreeable personalities, physically beautiful and well-educated. I very much hope to teach them to follow the life that I have led.

Now, I often fail to understand why men with fine bodies and minds who are in their middle years don't, when they come down with sicknesses, start being self-controlled in their eating and drinking. Is it because they are ignorant of how it will benefit them? I can't imagine that they are such slaves of their appetites that they're unable to change. I'm not surprised that younger men refuse to live such a life, since they are usually guided by their strong passions. And they don't have much experience. But when a man has made it to forty or fifty, you'd think he had figured it out. He should have learned that stuffing his face is not the best idea, as many say it is, but rather is the cause of sickness and death. And if the pleasure of eating and drinking heavily lasted, that would explain it. But the pleasures of gluttony and drunkenness are only momentary, compared to the duration of the diseases that such living causes.

THE THIRD DISCOURSE: ENJOYING HAPPINESS IN OLD AGE

My Lord,

When writing you, it's true that I'll be speaking of only a few things that I've already written to you about. But even though I've mentioned them in my essays, I'm sure that your Lordship won't tire of the repetition.

My Lord, To begin, I have to say that being 91 years old, I'm more sound and hearty than ever, much to the amazement of everyone who know me. I, who can account for this fact, am going to show that a person can enjoy an earthly paradise after eighty, but also that it can't be had without strict self-control with food and drink, virtues which God and friends appreciate. I need to tell you, though, that a lot of distinguished doctors from the university have visited me in the past few days, along with other doctors and philosophers who are well acquainted with my age, life, manners, as well as the fact that I'm stout, hearty and lively, with perfect senses, voice, teeth, memory and judgement. They also knew that I work eight hours a day in writing essays that are useful to mankind with my own hand, and also that I spend a lot of time walking and singing. Ih, my Lord, how beautiful my voice has grown! If you heard me chant my prayers on my lyre, just as David did, I'm sure that you would love it.

Now, these doctors and philosophers told me that it was next to a miracle that a man my age should be able to write about subjects that required both judgement and spirit. They added that I shouldn't be thought of as old, because the things I do every day are the same things that young men do. They said that I am completely unlike people in their seventies and eighties who have all sorts of ailments and diseases which make them weary. They also said that even if these old folks escape such things, their senses are impaired and that their sight, hearing, or memory is defective as are all of their other faculties. They aren't strong or cheerful as I am and they said that I have a special gift of grace along with telling me many great, eloquent, fine things while trying to prove this, which they couldn't because their comments weren't grounded on good and sufficient reasons, but merely their opinions. So I tried to set them straight and convince them that my happiness wasn't confined jut to me but could be common to all of humanity since I was a human being, no different from anyone else except for the fact that I was born weaker than some people, and not as strong as some are. The young, however, are prone to be led by sexual urges than reason, but when they reach forty or earlier, they should remember that they have reached the hilltop and must now think about going back down as they carry the weight of the years with them. I said that old age is the reverse of youth, just like order is the reverse of disorder, so it only makes sense that they should change their habits with regard to the quality and quantity of their food and drink. For isn't not possible that someone who is determined to stuff their face should be healthy and free from ailments. So to avoid this vice and its evil effects, I started controlling my intake of food and drink. It's true that I had a rough time doing this at the beginning, but I prayed to the Almighty to help me make that difficult change, and I knew that He would hear my prayer. Then I realized that someone can achieve a difficult goal if they set their mind to it, so I gradually let go of the excessive eating and drinking and began to take control over my intake. Before long, the sober and moderate life was no longer difficult, but I still made sure that I followed some very strict rules about the quantity and quality of the food I ate and drank.

Others who are blessed with stronger bodies can eat a lot more different foods than I, since each man is different from each other and can decide what food and drink suit him best. After he's found what he can take in, he should stick to that plan because he won't benefit much from it if he indulges in excess eating and drinking from time to time.

Now, when the doctors and philosophers heard all of this, they agreed that I had spoken the truth. One of the younger ones said that it looked as if it had been easy for me to trade my old life for the new one, and that it was easier than it sounded. He said that it was as difficult for him as it was easy for me.

I told him that since I'm human, it was no easy task for me but that I did it anyway because it wasn't manly for a man to lack courage to do a great and practical thing just because it was hard to do. The greater the obstacle to overcome, the greater the honor and benefit when it was accomplished. Our generous Creator wants us to live a long time, as He originally planned so that when we are past seventy, we can be finished with sexual lusts and govern ourselves with reason instead.

Wicked behavior and immorality leave and God is willing that he should live the full amount of years that was planned for him to live and that when this happens they should end their days without sickness but simply by dissolution, or to put it another way, fading comfortably away like a lamp that has run out of oil. This is the natural way for people to pass from this life. It's the wheels of life stopping quietly and a person peacefully leaving this world and going into immorality, which I will do some day, for I am sure to die in this way, maybe while I'm chanting my prayers. And thoughts of death don't give me the leas concern, neither does any other thought that's connected with death, namely the fear of punishment which wicked people may go to, because I am bound to believe that being a Christian, I shall be saved by the virtue of the most sacred blood of Jesus Christ which He freely shed to save those who trust in Him. So how beautiful is my life! How happy is my end! To this the young doctor had no reply except that he would follow my example.

The great desire I had, my Lord, to speak with you from this distance, has made me be too long-winded and wordy in my writing, and it still makes me write even more, but not much more. There are some people who live for their appetites, my Lord, who say that I have wasted my time by writing an essay on self-control and other things like it. They've said that it's impossible to do what I say and that I'll have little good come from my writing, much like "Plato on Government" who put a lot of effort in recommending something that wasn't doable. Now this is a really surprising because these people can see that I've lived a sober life for many years before I wrote about it. I would have never written about it if I hadn't been convinced that it was the right way to live. It's a true and wonderful life that would be of great service to these people if they would follow it. I felt the obligation to show it in its true light. Once again, I am thrilled to hear that many, upon reading my treatise, have followed what I've said. So the objection concerning Plato on Government does not stand up against what I say. But those people who live by their appetites are the enemy of reason and slaves to their passions.

THE FOURTH DISCOURSE: ENCOURAGEMENT TO LIVE TO OLD AGE

So that I won't be lacking in my duty or lose the satisfaction that I feel in being useful to others, I'm writing again to inform people who, since they can't speak directly with me, are strangers to the things that my immediate associates know and see. And while some of these things I say may seem incredible (even though they are true) I won't fail to still tell it for the public's benefit. So, I say, that being now at my ninety-fifth year, thank God, and still finding myself healthy and hearty, content and cheerful, I never stop thanking God for such blessings, when I consider the usual condition of old men. These usually don't make it to seventy without losing their health and spirts and growing depressed and sickly. Also, when I remember how weak and sickly I was between the ages of thirty and forty, and how from the first I never had a strong body, I must say that when I remember these things, I have a lot of cause for gratitude. And although I know that I can't live many more years, I have no problem with at the thought of dying. And further, I am certain that I'll live to be one hundred years. But to make this writing more organized, I'll start by considering people at their birth and then take them through every stage of life to the grave.

So I say that some people come into the world with such little strength that they only live a few days, months, or years. It's not always easy to tell why they are so weak. Others are born well but they still have poor, weak health. Of these, some live to the age of ten, twenty, thirty, or forty, but they seldom live to old age. Still others come into this world with perfect health and then make it to old age but as I've said, it's usually an old age of sickness and sorrow which they can only blame on themselves, since they took their good health for granted. And by the time they're old, they can't change from the life they've lived through the years, and they continue to live as excessively as they did when they were young when they've passed the full circle of their lives. They don't realize that their stomachs have lost much of its natural heat and energy and that they should pay strict attention to the quality and quantity of what they eat and drink. But rather than decrease their intake, many of them increase it and they say that as their health and energy decrease, the need to repair the loss by stuffing themselves, because they think that such eating preserves us.

But this is where they make their great mistake, because as their body's energy and heat decreases with old age, they should decrease their food and drink because nature, in old age, is content with little. Also, if increasing their food was the right thing to do, then most people would live to old age with good health. But do we see that happening? No. Such cases are rare exceptions, while my course of life has proved to be the right way, since the results are easy to see. But even though some people can see my results, because of their lack of personality strength and their love of uncontrolled eating and drinking, they still continue to eat and drink the way they've always done. If, on the other hand, they formed strict, self-controlled habits, they wouldn't grow sickly in their old age but would be, as I am, strong and hearty and might live to the age of one hundred or one hundred and twenty. This has happened to others that we read about, people who were born with good health and lived sober, self-controlled lives. And had I been born with good health, I would probably make it to that age. But since I was born feeble and with sickly health, I'm afraid that I won't outlive one hundred years. And if there are others that were born weak like me, if they lived a life like mine, they would also live to one hundred as I will.

And being certain of living to an old age is, in my opinion, a great advantage (of course, I don't include accidents, which can happen to anyone, and which we must leave to our Maker), and should be highly valued. No one can be sure of this blessing except the ones that stick to the rules of self-control. This security of life is built on good, natural reasons which can't fail. It's impossible for anyone that leads a perfectly sober and self-controlled life to breed any sicknesses or die before their time. Also, such a person can't die from sickness because such a sober life has the power to remove whatever causes sickness, and sickness can't happen without a cause. So when the cause is removed, sickness is also removed and untimely and painful death is prevented.

And there's no doubt that self-control in food and drink, taking only as much as nature really requires (and being guided by reason instead of appetite), has the ability to remove all causes of disease. For since health and sickness, life and death, depend on the good or bad condition of a person's blood and the quality of his other fluids, this life that I describe purifies the blood and corrects all dangerous fluids and makes them all perfect and harmonious. It's true and can't be denied that a person must finally die, no matter how careful they've been. But I maintain that it will be without sickness and great pain. In my case I expect to pass away quietly and peacefully, and my present condition insures that this will happen. And even though I'm at a great age, I'm strong and content, eating with a good appetite and sleeping soundly. Further, all of my senses are as good as ever and in the best condition. My understanding is clear and bright, my judgement sound, my memory firm, my spirits good, and my voice (which is one of the first things that usually fails us) has grown so strong and full, that I can't help chanting my prayers out loud in the morning and the night, instead of whispering and muttering them to myself as I used to do.

Oh how glorious is this life of mine, filled with all of the abilities to express myself that a man can enjoy on this side of the grave! It's completely lacking from the sexual brutality, which age has allowed my reason to get rid of. So I'm not troubled with passions and my mind is calm and free from all worries and doubtful concerns. And there's no room in my mind for thinking of death, at least, not in a way that disturbs me. And all of this has been brought about, by God's mercy, through my careful habit of living. How different it is from the life of most old men, which are full of aches and pains and dread, while mine is a life of real pleasure and I spend my days in fun pursuits as I'll soon show.

First, I am of service to my country. This is a joy. It's infinitely delightful to work on different improvements on the mouth of the river or the harbor of this city and fortifications. And although this Venice, this Queen of the Sea, is very beautiful and wealthier, since I've shown how she can have a lot of provisions. I've improved large tracts of land and converted marshes and barren sand to farmland. Also, I have another joy that's always present with me. Some time ago I lost a lot of my income, which would have negatively affected my grandchildren. But I, by thinking things through, have found a true and perfect method of repairing such loss by more than double, by the sensible use of that recommendable art known as agriculture. Another great comfort to me is to think that my writing on self-control is really useful, as many people have verbally told me as well as written. They say that under God, they are indebted to me for their lives. It's also a pleasure to write and be of service to myself and others. It gives me a lot of pleasure to talk with able men who have superior understanding, who teach me new things. Now, what a comfort that, as old as I am, I'm able, without getting tired in my mind or body, to be fully engaged to study the most important, difficult, and excellent subjects.

I need to further add that at this age, I seem to be enjoying two lives: one here on the earth, which I actually possess, and the other one, which is heavenly, which I possess in thought. And this thought is really enjoyable since it's founded on things that we are certain to get some day. And I'm certain, by the infinite goodness of God that I will receive eternal life. So, I enjoy life on earth as a result of my sobriety and self-control (virtues that are agreeable to God), and I also enjoy, by the grace of God, the heavenly, which He causes me to anticipate in my thoughts. And it's a lively thought that keeps my attention, since I know with certainty that I'll eventually live in Heaven. And I maintain that dying in the manner that I expect to die isn't really death, but a passage of the soul from this earthly life to a heavenly, immortal, and infinitely perfect existence. It can't be any other way and this thought is so pleasing and above all else and excellent that it is far above all worldly thoughts such as the death of this body, since my thoughts are focused on the happiness of living a heavenly and divine life. So it is that I enjoy two lives, and the thought of ending this earthly life gives me no worry, because I know that I have a glorious and immortal life before me.

Now, is it possible that anyone should grow tired of such a great comfort and blessing as this that I enjoy and which most people can also have, simply by leading the life that I've led, which is an example that everyone is able to follow? I'm no saint but rather a mere man and a servant of God to whom a regular, consistent life works very well.

Now there are people who embrace a spiritual and contemplative life, and this is holy and commendable. Their chief activity is to celebrate the praises of God and to teach men how to serve Him. How, if while these men set themselves apart for such a life, they would also set out to living sober and self-controlled lives, how much more agreeable would they cause themselves to be in God's sight and the sight of men? How much greater could they honor and decorate this world? They would at the same time enjoy constant health and happiness, would live to an old age, and as a result become famously wise and useful, whereas now, they are mostly sick, grumpy and unsatisfied. They think that their different trials and sicknesses are sent to them by Almighty God, so that He can promote their salvation by giving them a punishment in this life for their past errors. Now, I can't help saying that in my opinion they are greatly mistaken. For I can't believe that God desires humans, who are his favorite creatures, to be sick and depressed but rather, that they should enjoy good health and happiness. But people bring sickness and disease on themselves either through ignorance or willful self-indulgence. Now, if those who say they are our teachers about God would set an example for the rest of us and teach people how to preserve their bodies with health, they would do a lot to make the road to Heaven easier. People need to be taught that self-denial and strict self-control is the path to health of body and mind, and those who live this way see more clearly than others as to what their duty is toward our Savior Jesus Christ, who came down to earth to shed His precious blood so that we could be delivered from the tyranny of the devil. This was His hue goodness and loving kindness to humanity.

Now, to end this writing, I say that since my years are so full of favors and blessings, and I, not by theory but by happy experience can verify it, I sincerely assure everyone that I really enjoy a lot more than I can mention, and that I have no other reason for writing but to demonstrate the great advantages that come from living a long time, and living such a life as I've lived. It's my desire to convince people to follow these excellent rules of constant self-control in eating and drinking. So for this reason I don't ever stop raising my voice and crying out to you, my friends, so that your lives may be even as mine.

About the Author

Luigi Cornaro was born in 1467. He was a Venetian nobleman and patron of the arts. When he was between 35 and 40, he found himself exhausted and in poor health, a condition he attributed to his hedonistic lifestyle with over eating, drinking, and sexual excesses. His doctors instructed him to change his lifestyle or he would be dead in a year. Taking their advice, he had immediate results and within that year all of his symptoms disappeared. He wrote four books on self-control and health (published between 1583–95) which detailed his secrets on living with good health to a ripe old age. He died in 1569 at the age of 102.

About the Editor

George (G.U.) Steffner is a fifth-generation native of Atlanta, Georgia and he is a graduate of The Citadel in Charleston, South Carolina where he earned a degree in English. After a brief stint at Fort Bragg, he chased bad guys through Atlanta's most exclusive stores, joined a cult, flipped burgers at several fast food restaurants, occupied a skyscraper's corner office in a large law firm, and nailed-down and refinished hardwood floors all over the Southeastern United States. He writes under several different pen names and lives in Atlanta with his enormous family and his leather-lunged hound dogs.